Yoga Teacher Planner

This notebook BELONGS TO

....

DATE

....

If found, please return to

....

"Inhale the future, exhale the past."

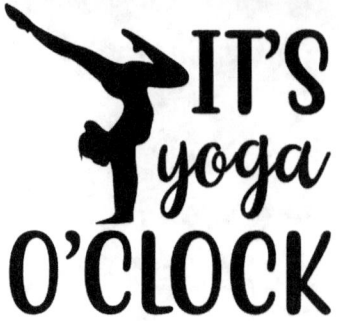

YOGA MONTHLY PLANNER

MONTH:

MON	TUE	WED	THU	FRI	SAT	SUN

GOALS:

NOTES:

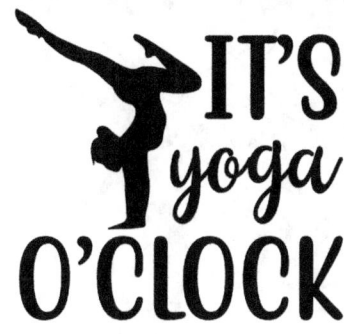

YOGA MONTHLY PLANNER

MONTH:

MON	TUE	WED	THU	FRI	SAT	SUN

GOALS:

NOTES:

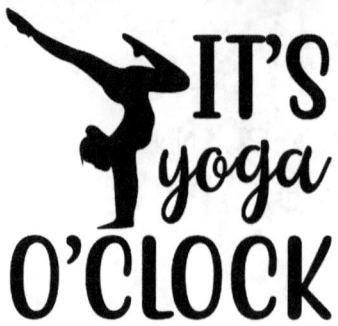

YOGA MONTHLY PLANNER

MONTH:

MON	TUE	WED	THU	FRI	SAT	SUN

GOALS:

NOTES:

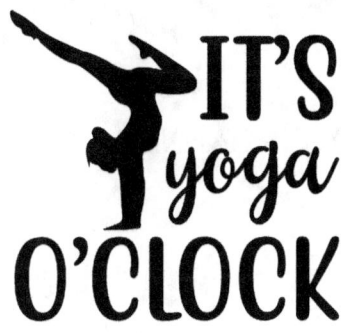

YOGA MONTHLY PLANNER

MONTH:

MON	TUE	WED	THU	FRI	SAT	SUN

GOALS:

NOTES:

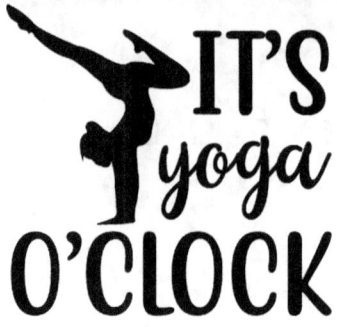

YOGA MONTHLY PLANNER
MONTH:

MON	TUE	WED	THU	FRI	SAT	SUN

GOALS:

NOTES:

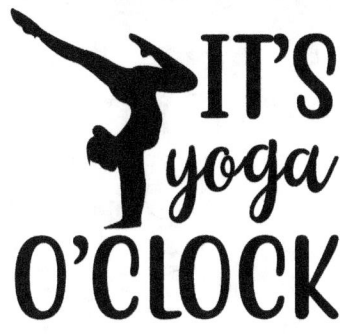

YOGA MONTHLY PLANNER

MONTH:

MON	TUE	WED	THU	FRI	SAT	SUN

GOALS:

NOTES:

index

Page no

index

Page no

index

Page no

"It's not about being good at something. It's about being good to yourself."

Yoga Teacher Planner

Date

Time

Venue

Theme/Focus:

Props

Oils

Music

No. Of Attendees:

Private class: y / n

Note
-
-
-
-
-
-
-
-
-

Feedback

☆ ☆ ☆ ☆ ☆

Mantra / Positive Quote:

Important facts to remember

All my notes sequencing

Yoga Teacher Planner

Date

Time

Venue

Theme/Focus:

Props

Oils   Music

No. Of Attendees:

Private class: y / n

Note
-
-
-
-
-
-
-
-
-

Feedback

☆ ☆ ☆ ☆ ☆

Mantra / Positive Quote:

Important facts to remember:

All my notes sequencing

Yoga Teacher Planner

Date
Time
Venue

Theme/Focus:

Props

Oils   Music

No. Of Attendees:
Private class: y / n

Note

○
○
○
○
○
○
○
○

Feedback

☆ ☆ ☆ ☆ ☆

Mantra / Positive Quote:

Important facts to remember:

....
....
....
....

All my notes sequencing

Yoga Teacher Planner

Date

Time

Venue

Theme/Focus:

Props

Oils

Music

No. Of Attendees:

Private class: y / n

Note

-
-
-
-
-
-
-
-
-

Feedback

☆ ☆ ☆ ☆ ☆

Mantra / Positive Quote:

Important facts to remember

....

....

....

....

All my notes sequencing

Yoga Teacher Planner

Date

Time

Venue

Theme/Focus:

Props

Oils

Music

No. Of Attendees:

Private class: y / n

Note

-
-
-
-
-
-
-
-

Feedback

☆ ☆ ☆ ☆ ☆

Mantra / Positive Quote:

Important facts to remember:

All my notes sequencing

Yoga Teacher Planner

Date

Time

Venue

Theme/Focus:

Props

Oils

Music

No. Of Attendees:

Private class: y / n

Note

○
○
○
○
○
○
○
○

Feedback

☆ ☆ ☆ ☆ ☆

Mantra / Positive Quote:

Important facts to remember:

All my notes sequencing

Yoga Teacher Planner

Date

Time

Venue

Theme/Focus:

Props

Oils

Music

No. Of Attendees:

Private class: y / n

Note
-
-
-
-
-
-
-
-

Feedback

☆ ☆ ☆ ☆ ☆

Mantra / Positive Quote:

Important facts to remember

All my notes sequencing

Yoga Teacher Planner

Date

Time

Venue

Theme/Focus:

Props

Oils

Music

No. Of Attendees:

Private class: y / n

Note
-
-
-
-
-
-
-
-
-

Feedback

☆ ☆ ☆ ☆ ☆

Mantra / Positive Quote:

Important facts to remember:

....

....

....

....

All my notes sequencing

Yoga Teacher Planner

Date

Time

Venue

Theme/Focus:

Props

Oils

Music

No. Of Attendees:

Private class: y / n

Note

-
-
-
-
-
-
-
-

Feedback

☆ ☆ ☆ ☆ ☆

Mantra / Positive Quote:

Important facts to remember:

....

....

....

....

All my notes sequencing

Yoga Teacher Planner

Date

Time

Venue

Theme/Focus:

Props

Oils

Music

No. Of Attendees:

Private class: y / n

Note
-
-
-
-
-
-
-
-
-

Feedback

☆ ☆ ☆ ☆ ☆

Mantra / Positive Quote:

Important facts to remember:

....

....

....

....

All my notes sequencing

"Be where you are, not where you think you should be."

Yoga Teacher Planner

Date

Time

Venue

Theme/Focus:

Props

Oils   Music

No. Of Attendees:

Private class: y / n

Note
-
-
-
-
-
-
-
-

Feedback

☆ ☆ ☆ ☆ ☆

Mantra / Positive Quote:

Important facts to remember

All my notes sequencing

Yoga Teacher Planner

Date

Time

Venue

Theme/Focus:

Props

Oils

Music

No. Of Attendees:

Private class: y / n

Note

-
-
-
-
-
-
-
-

Feedback

☆ ☆ ☆ ☆ ☆

Mantra / Positive Quote:

Important facts to remember:

All my notes sequencing

Yoga Teacher Planner

Date

Time

Venue

Theme/Focus:

Props

Oils

Music

No. Of Attendees:

Private class: y / n

Note

-
-
-
-
-
-
-
-
-

Feedback

☆ ☆ ☆ ☆ ☆

Mantra / Positive Quote:

Important facts to remember:

All my notes sequencing

Yoga Teacher Planner

Date

Time

Venue

Theme/Focus:

Props

Oils　　　　　　　Music

No. Of Attendees:

Private class:　y / n

Note

-
-
-
-
-
-
-
-

Feedback

☆ ☆ ☆ ☆ ☆

Mantra / Positive Quote:

Important facts to remember:

....

....

....

....

All my notes sequencing

Yoga Teacher Planner

Date

Time

Venue

Theme/Focus:

Props

Oils

Music

No. Of Attendees:

Private class: y / n

Note
-
-
-
-
-
-
-
-

Feedback

☆ ☆ ☆ ☆ ☆

Mantra / Positive Quote:

Important facts to remember:

All my notes sequencing

Yoga Teacher Planner

Date

Time

Venue

Theme/Focus:

Props

Oils   Music

No. Of Attendees:

Private class: y / n

Note

-
-
-
-
-
-
-
-

Feedback

☆ ☆ ☆ ☆ ☆

Mantra / Positive Quote:

Important facts to remember:

All my notes sequencing

Yoga Teacher Planner

Date

Time

Venue

Theme/Focus:

Props

Oils

Music

No. Of Attendees:

Private class: y / n

Note

○
○
○
○
○
○
○
○

Feedback

☆ ☆ ☆ ☆ ☆

Mantra / Positive Quote:

Important facts to remember

All my notes sequencing

Yoga Teacher Planner

Date

Time

Venue

Theme/Focus:

Props

Oils

Music

No. Of Attendees:

Private class: y / n

Note

-
-
-
-
-
-
-
-

Feedback

☆ ☆ ☆ ☆ ☆

Mantra / Positive Quote:

Important facts to remember:

All my notes sequencing

Yoga Teacher Planner

Date

Time

Venue

Theme/Focus:

Props

Oils

Music

No. Of Attendees:

Private class: y / n

Note
-
-
-
-
-
-
-
-
-

Feedback

☆ ☆ ☆ ☆ ☆

Mantra / Positive Quote:

Important facts to remember:

....

....

....

....

All my notes sequencing

Yoga Teacher Planner

Date

Time

Venue

Theme/Focus:

Props

Oils

Music

No. Of Attendees:

Private class: y / n

Note
-
-
-
-
-
-
-
-

Feedback

☆ ☆ ☆ ☆ ☆

Mantra / Positive Quote:

Important facts to remember

....

....

....

....

All my notes sequencing

"Inhale the future, exhale the past."

Yoga Teacher Planner

Date

Time

Venue

Theme/Focus:

Props

Oils

Music

No. Of Attendees:

Private class: y / n

Note

○
○
○
○
○
○
○
○
○

Feedback

☆ ☆ ☆ ☆ ☆

Mantra / Positive Quote:

Important facts to remember:

All my notes sequencing

Yoga Teacher Planner

Date

Time

Venue

Theme/Focus:

Props

Oils

Music

No. Of Attendees:

Private class: y / n

Note

-
-
-
-
-
-
-
-

Feedback

☆ ☆ ☆ ☆ ☆

Mantra / Positive Quote:

Important facts to remember:

....

....

....

....

All my notes sequencing

Yoga Teacher Planner

Date

Time

Venue

Theme/Focus:

Props

Oils   Music

No. Of Attendees:

Private class: y / n

Note
-
-
-
-
-
-
-
-
-

Feedback

☆ ☆ ☆ ☆ ☆

Mantra / Positive Quote:

Important facts to remember:

All my notes sequencing

Yoga Teacher Planner

Date

Time

Venue

Theme/Focus:

Props

Oils

Music

No. Of Attendees:

Private class: y / n

Note

○
○
○
○
○
○
○
○
○

Feedback

☆ ☆ ☆ ☆ ☆

Mantra / Positive Quote:

Important facts to remember

All my notes sequencing

Yoga Teacher Planner

Date

Time

Venue

Theme/Focus:

Props

Oils

Music

No. Of Attendees:

Private class: y / n

Note

-
-
-
-
-
-
-
-

Feedback

☆ ☆ ☆ ☆ ☆

Mantra / Positive Quote:

Important facts to remember:

All my notes sequencing

Yoga Teacher Planner

Date

Time

Venue

Theme/Focus:

Props

Oils   Music

No. Of Attendees:

Private class: y / n

Note

○ _____
○ _____
○ _____
○ _____
○ _____
○ _____
○ _____
○ _____
○ _____

Feedback

☆ ☆ ☆ ☆ ☆

Mantra / Positive Quote:

Important facts to remember:

....

....

....

....

All my notes sequencing

Yoga Teacher Planner

Date

Time

Venue

Theme/Focus:

Props

Oils　　　　　　　　Music

No. Of Attendees:

Private class:　y / n

Note

-
-
-
-
-
-
-
-

Feedback

☆ ☆ ☆ ☆ ☆

Mantra / Positive Quote:

Important facts to remember

All my notes sequencing

Yoga Teacher Planner

Date

Time

Venue

Theme/Focus:

Props

Oils   Music

No. Of Attendees:

Private class: y / n

Note

-
-
-
-
-
-
-
-

Feedback

☆ ☆ ☆ ☆ ☆

Mantra / Positive Quote:

Important facts to remember:

All my notes sequencing

Yoga Teacher Planner

Date

Time

Venue

Theme/Focus:

Props

Oils   Music

No. Of Attendees:

Private class: y / n

Note

○
○
○
○
○
○
○
○
○

Feedback

☆ ☆ ☆ ☆ ☆

Mantra / Positive Quote:

Important facts to remember:

....

....

....

....

All my notes sequencing

Yoga Teacher Planner

Date

Time

Venue

Theme/Focus:

Props

Oils

Music

No. Of Attendees:

Private class: y / n

Note
-
-
-
-
-
-
-
-

Feedback

☆ ☆ ☆ ☆ ☆

Mantra / Positive Quote:

Important facts to remember:

All my notes sequencing

"The pose begins when you want to leave it."

Yoga Teacher Planner

Date

Time

Venue

Theme/Focus:

Props

Oils   Music

No. Of Attendees:

Private class: y / n

Note
-
-
-
-
-
-
-
-

Feedback

☆ ☆ ☆ ☆ ☆

Mantra / Positive Quote:

Important facts to remember:

....

....

....

....

All my notes sequencing

Yoga Teacher Planner

Date

Time

Venue

Theme/Focus:

Props

Oils

Music

No. Of Attendees:

Private class: y / n

Note

○
○
○
○
○
○
○
○

Feedback

☆ ☆ ☆ ☆ ☆

Mantra / Positive Quote:

Important facts to remember:

All my notes sequencing

Yoga Teacher Planner

Date

Time

Venue

Theme/Focus:

Props

Oils

Music

No. Of Attendees:

Private class: y / n

Note

-
-
-
-
-
-
-
-
-

Feedback

☆ ☆ ☆ ☆ ☆

Mantra / Positive Quote:

Important facts to remember

All my notes sequencing

Yoga Teacher Planner

Date

Time

Venue

Theme/Focus:

Props

Oils

Music

No. Of Attendees:

Private class: y / n

Note

○
○
○
○
○
○
○
○

Feedback

☆ ☆ ☆ ☆ ☆

Mantra / Positive Quote:

Important facts to remember:

All my notes sequencing

Yoga Teacher Planner

Date

Time

Venue

Theme/Focus:

Props

Oils

Music

No. Of Attendees:

Private class: y / n

Note

-
-
-
-
-
-
-
-

Feedback

☆ ☆ ☆ ☆ ☆

Mantra / Positive Quote:

Important facts to remember:

....

....

....

....

All my notes sequencing

Yoga Teacher Planner

Date

Time

Venue

Theme/Focus:

Props

Oils

Music

No. Of Attendees:

Private class: y / n

Note
-
-
-
-
-
-
-
-

Feedback

☆ ☆ ☆ ☆ ☆

Mantra / Positive Quote:

Important facts to remember:

All my notes sequencing

Yoga Teacher Planner

Date
Time
Venue

Theme/Focus:

Props

Oils

Music

No. Of Attendees:
Private class: y / n

Note
-
-
-
-
-
-
-
-
-

Feedback

☆ ☆ ☆ ☆ ☆

Mantra / Positive Quote:

Important facts to remember:

....
....
....
....

All my notes sequencing

Yoga Teacher Planner

Date

Time

Venue

Theme/Focus:

Props

Oils   Music

No. Of Attendees:

Private class: y / n

Note

-
-
-
-
-
-
-
-
-

Feedback

☆ ☆ ☆ ☆ ☆

Mantra / Positive Quote:

Important facts to remember:

....

....

....

....

All my notes sequencing

Yoga Teacher Planner

Date

Time

Venue

Theme/Focus:

Props

Oils

Music

No. Of Attendees:

Private class: y / n

Note

○
○
○
○
○
○
○
○

Feedback

☆ ☆ ☆ ☆ ☆

Mantra / Positive Quote:

Important facts to remember:

All my notes sequencing

Yoga Teacher Planner

Date

Time

Venue

Theme/Focus:

Props

Oils

Music

No. Of Attendees:

Private class: y / n

Note
-
-
-
-
-
-
-
-

Feedback

☆ ☆ ☆ ☆ ☆

Mantra / Positive Quote:

Important facts to remember

....

....

....

....

All my notes sequencing

"*Letting go is the hardest asana.*"

Yoga Teacher Planner

Date

Time

Venue

Theme/Focus:

Props

Oils

Music

No. Of Attendees:

Private class: y / n

Note

○
○
○
○
○
○
○
○
○

Feedback

☆ ☆ ☆ ☆ ☆

Mantra / Positive Quote:

Important facts to remember:

All my notes sequencing

Yoga Teacher Planner

Date

Time

Venue

Theme/Focus:

Props

Oils

Music

No. Of Attendees:

Private class: y / n

Note

○
○
○
○
○
○
○
○

Feedback

☆ ☆ ☆ ☆ ☆

Mantra / Positive Quote:

Important facts to remember:

All my notes sequencing

Yoga Teacher Planner

Date

Time

Venue

Theme/Focus:

Props

Oils   Music

No. Of Attendees:

Private class: y / n

Note
-
-
-
-
-
-
-
-
-

Feedback

☆ ☆ ☆ ☆ ☆

Mantra / Positive Quote:

Important facts to remember

....

....

....

....

All my notes sequencing

Yoga Teacher Planner

Date

Time

Venue

Theme/Focus:

Props

Oils

Music

No. Of Attendees:

Private class: y / n

Note

-
-
-
-
-
-
-
-
-

Feedback

☆ ☆ ☆ ☆ ☆

Mantra / Positive Quote:

Important facts to remember

All my notes sequencing

Yoga Teacher Planner

Date

Time

Venue

Theme/Focus:

Props

Oils

Music

No. Of Attendees:

Private class: y / n

Note
-
-
-
-
-
-
-
-
-
-

Feedback

☆ ☆ ☆ ☆ ☆

Mantra / Positive Quote:

Important facts to remember

All my notes sequencing

Yoga Teacher Planner

Date

Time

Venue

Theme/Focus:

Props

Oils

Music

No. Of Attendees:

Private class: y / n

Note

-
-
-
-
-
-
-
-
-

Feedback

☆ ☆ ☆ ☆ ☆

Mantra / Positive Quote:

Important facts to remember:

All my notes sequencing

Yoga Teacher Planner

Date

Time

Venue

Theme/Focus:

Props

Oils

Music

No. Of Attendees:

Private class: y / n

Note

-
-
-
-
-
-
-
-
-

Feedback

☆ ☆ ☆ ☆ ☆

Mantra / Positive Quote:

Important facts to remember

All my notes sequencing

Yoga Teacher Planner

Date

Time

Venue

Theme/Focus:

Props

Oils

Music

No. Of Attendees:

Private class: y / n

Note
-
-
-
-
-
-
-
-
-

Feedback

☆ ☆ ☆ ☆ ☆

Mantra / Positive Quote:

Important facts to remember:

....

....

....

....

All my notes sequencing

Yoga Teacher Planner

Date

Time

Venue

Theme/Focus:

Props

Oils

Music

No. Of Attendees:

Private class: y / n

Note
-
-
-
-
-
-
-
-

Feedback

☆ ☆ ☆ ☆ ☆

Mantra / Positive Quote:

Important facts to remember:

....
....
....
....

All my notes sequencing

Yoga Teacher Planner

Date

Time

Venue

Theme/Focus:

Props

Oils

Music

No. Of Attendees:

Private class: y / n

Note
-
-
-
-
-
-
-
-
-

Feedback

☆ ☆ ☆ ☆ ☆

Mantra / Positive Quote:

Important facts to remember

....

....

....

....

All my notes sequencing

"A flower does not think of competing to the flower next to it. It just blooms."

Yoga Teacher Planner

Date

Time

Venue

Theme/Focus:

Props

Oils

Music

No. Of Attendees:

Private class: y / n

Note
-
-
-
-
-
-
-
-

Feedback

☆ ☆ ☆ ☆ ☆

Mantra / Positive Quote:

Important facts to remember

....

....

....

....

All my notes sequencing

Yoga Teacher Planner

Date
Time
Venue

Theme/Focus:

Props

Oils

Music

No. Of Attendees:

Private class: y / n

Note
-
-
-
-
-
-
-
-

Feedback

☆ ☆ ☆ ☆ ☆

Mantra / Positive Quote:

Important facts to remember

All my notes sequencing

Yoga Teacher Planner

Date

Time

Venue

Theme/Focus:

Props

Oils

Music

No. Of Attendees:

Private class: y / n

Note
-
-
-
-
-
-
-
-

Feedback

☆ ☆ ☆ ☆ ☆

Mantra / Positive Quote:

Important facts to remember

All my notes sequencing

Yoga Teacher Planner

Date

Time

Venue

Theme/Focus:

Props
....
....
....
....
....
....
....
....
....
....

Oils

Music

No. Of Attendees:

Private class: y / n

Note
○ _____
○ _____
○ _____
○ _____
○ _____
○ _____
○ _____
○ _____

Feedback

☆ ☆ ☆ ☆ ☆

Mantra / Positive Quote:

Important facts to remember

....
....
....
....

All my notes sequencing

Yoga Teacher Planner

Date

Time

Venue

Theme/Focus:

Props

Oils   Music

No. Of Attendees:

Private class: y / n

Note
-
-
-
-
-
-
-
-

Feedback

☆ ☆ ☆ ☆ ☆

Mantra / Positive Quote:

Important facts to remember:

All my notes sequencing

Yoga Teacher Planner

Date

Time

Venue

Theme/Focus:

Props

Oils   Music

No. Of Attendees:

Private class: y / n

Note

○
○
○
○
○
○
○
○

Feedback

☆ ☆ ☆ ☆ ☆

Mantra / Positive Quote:

Important facts to remember:

All my notes sequencing

Yoga Teacher Planner

Date

Time

Venue

Theme/Focus:

Props ....
....
....
....
....
....
....
....

Oils   Music

No. Of Attendees:

Private class: y / n

Note

○ ──────────
○ ──────────
○ ──────────
○ ──────────
○ ──────────
○ ──────────
○ ──────────
○ ──────────

Feedback

☆ ☆ ☆ ☆ ☆

Mantra / Positive Quote:

Important facts to remember

....
....
....
....

All my notes sequencing

Yoga Teacher Planner

Date

Time

Venue

Theme/Focus:

Props

Oils

Music

No. Of Attendees:

Private class: y / n

Note
-
-
-
-
-
-
-
-

Feedback

☆ ☆ ☆ ☆ ☆

Mantra / Positive Quote:

Important facts to remember:

All my notes sequencing

Yoga Teacher Planner

Date

Time

Venue

Theme/Focus:

Props

Oils

Music

No. Of Attendees:

Private class: y / n

Note
-
-
-
-
-
-
-
-

Feedback

☆ ☆ ☆ ☆ ☆

Mantra / Positive Quote:

Important facts to remember:

....

....

....

....

All my notes sequencing

Yoga Teacher Planner

Date

Time

Venue

Theme/Focus:

Props

Oils

Music

No. Of Attendees:

Private class: y / n

Note

○
○
○
○
○
○
○
○

Feedback

☆ ☆ ☆ ☆ ☆

Mantra / Positive Quote:

Important facts to remember

....

....

....

....

All my notes sequencing

"Just breathe."

Yoga Teacher Planner

Date

Time

Venue

Theme/Focus:

Props

Oils

Music

No. Of Attendees:

Private class: y / n

Note

-
-
-
-
-
-
-
-
-

Feedback

☆ ☆ ☆ ☆ ☆

Mantra / Positive Quote:

Important facts to remember

....

....

....

....

All my notes sequencing

Yoga Teacher Planner

Date

Time

Venue

Theme/Focus:

Props

Oils

Music

No. Of Attendees:

Private class: y / n

Note

- _____
- _____
- _____
- _____
- _____
- _____
- _____
- _____
- _____

Feedback

☆ ☆ ☆ ☆ ☆

Mantra / Positive Quote:

Important facts to remember:

....

....

....

....

All my notes sequencing

Yoga Teacher Planner

Date

Time

Venue

Theme/Focus:

Props

Oils   Music

No. Of Attendees:

Private class: y / n

Note
-
-
-
-
-
-
-
-
-

Feedback

☆ ☆ ☆ ☆ ☆

Mantra / Positive Quote:

Important facts to remember:

....

....

....

....

All my notes sequencing

Yoga Teacher Planner

Date

Time

Venue

Theme/Focus:

Props

Oils   Music

No. Of Attendees:

Private class: y / n

Note
-
-
-
-
-
-
-
-

Feedback

☆ ☆ ☆ ☆ ☆

Mantra / Positive Quote:

Important facts to remember

All my notes sequencing

Yoga Teacher Planner

Date

Time

Venue

Theme/Focus:

Props

Oils

Music

No. Of Attendees:

Private class: y / n

Note

○
○
○
○
○
○
○
○
○

Feedback

☆ ☆ ☆ ☆ ☆

Mantra / Positive Quote:

Important facts to remember

All my notes sequencing

Yoga Teacher Planner

Date

Time

Venue

Theme/Focus:

Props

Oils

Music

No. Of Attendees:

Private class: y / n

Note

-
-
-
-
-
-
-
-
-

Feedback

☆ ☆ ☆ ☆ ☆

Mantra / Positive Quote:

Important facts to remember:

All my notes sequencing

Yoga Teacher Planner

Date

Time

Venue

Theme/Focus:

Props

Oils

Music

No. Of Attendees:

Private class: y / n

Note

○
○
○
○
○
○
○
○

Feedback

☆ ☆ ☆ ☆ ☆

Mantra / Positive Quote:

Important facts to remember:

All my notes sequencing

Yoga Teacher Planner

Date

Time

Venue

Theme/Focus:

Props

Oils

Music

No. Of Attendees:

Private class: y / n

Note
-
-
-
-
-
-
-
-

Feedback

☆ ☆ ☆ ☆ ☆

Mantra / Positive Quote:

Important facts to remember:

All my notes sequencing

Yoga Teacher Planner

Date

Time

Venue

Theme/Focus:

Props

Oils   Music

No. Of Attendees:

Private class: y / n

Note
-
-
-
-
-
-
-
-
-

Feedback

☆ ☆ ☆ ☆ ☆

Mantra / Positive Quote:

Important facts to remember

All my notes sequencing

Yoga Teacher Planner

Date

Time

Venue

Theme/Focus:

Props

Oils

Music

No. Of Attendees:

Private class: y / n

Note

-
-
-
-
-
-
-
-

Feedback

☆ ☆ ☆ ☆ ☆

Mantra / Positive Quote:

Important facts to remember

All my notes sequencing

30 Yoga Basic Poses

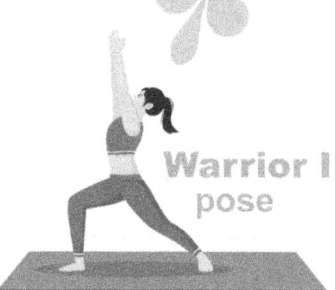
Warrior I pose

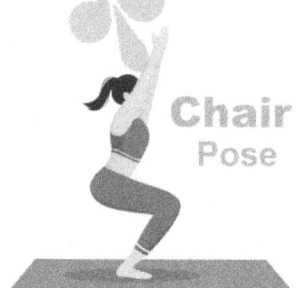
Chair Pose

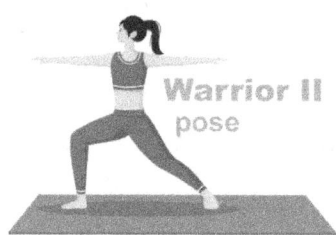
Warrior II pose

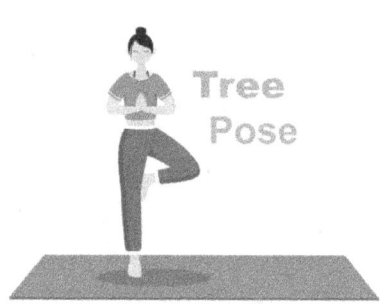
Tree Pose

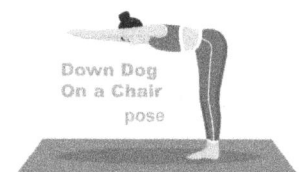
Down Dog On a Chair pose

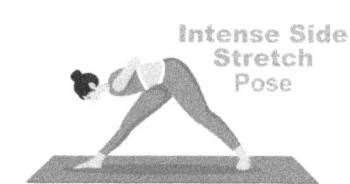
Intense Side Stretch Pose

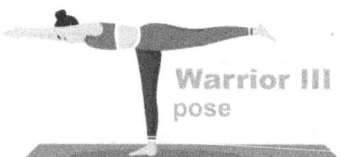
Warrior III pose

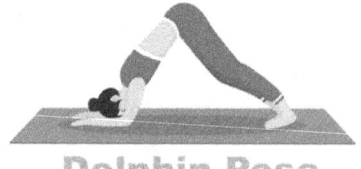
Dolphin Pose

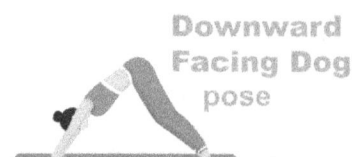
Downward Facing Dog pose

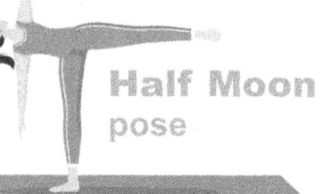
Half Moon pose

30 Yoga Basic Poses

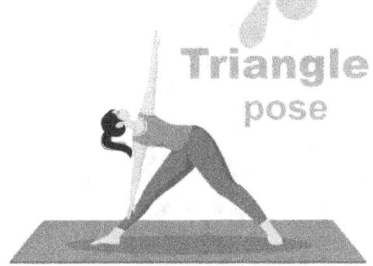
Triangle pose

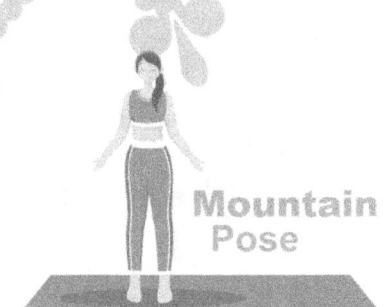
Mountain Pose

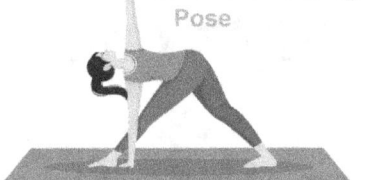
Revolved Triangle Pose

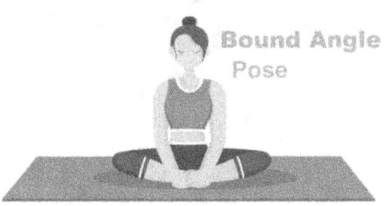
Bound Angle Pose

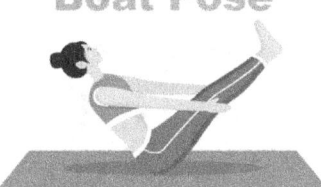
Boat Pose

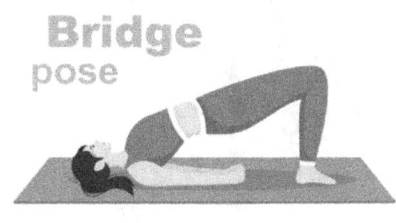
Bridge pose

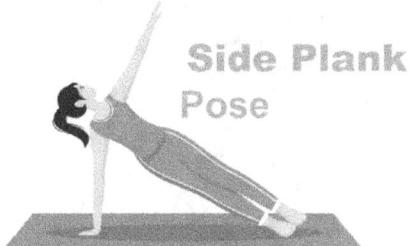
Side Plank Pose

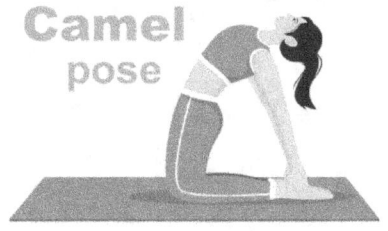
Camel pose

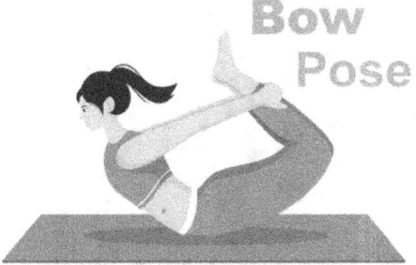
Bow Pose

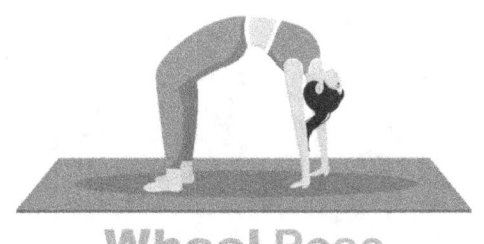
Wheel Pose

30 Yoga Basic Poses

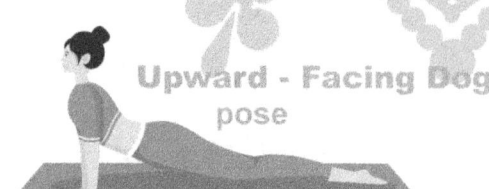
Upward - Facing Dog pose

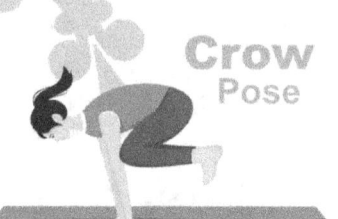
Crow Pose

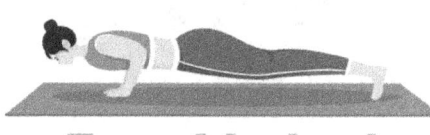
Four-Limbed Staff Pose

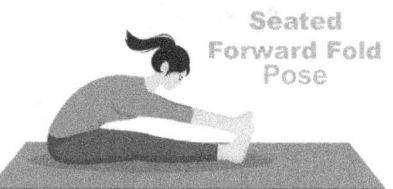
Seated Forward Fold Pose

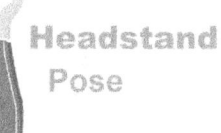
Headstand Pose

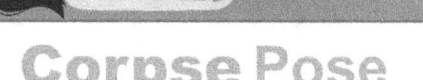
Corpse Pose

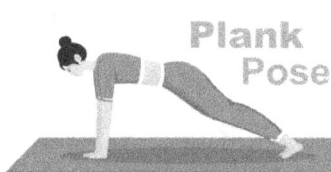
Plank Pose

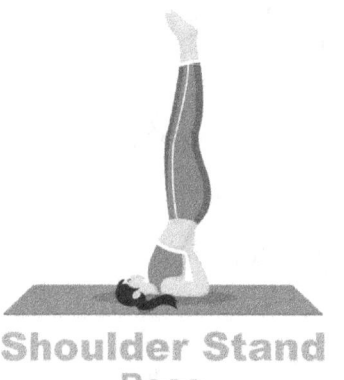
Shoulder Stand Pose

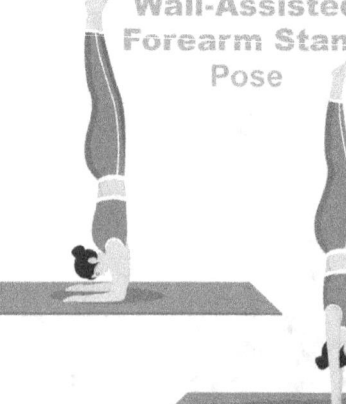
Wall-Assisted Forearm Stand Pose

Wall-Assisted Handstand Pose

Copyrights 2022 - All rights reserved

You may not reproduce, duplicate, or send the contents of this book without direct written permission from the author. You cannot hereby despite any circumstance blame the publisher or hold him or her the legal responsibility for any reparation, compensation or monetary forfeiture owing to the information included herein, either in a direct or indirect way.

Legal Notice: This book has copyright protection. You can use the book for personal purpose. You should not sell, use, alter, distribute, quote, take excerpts or paraphrase in part of whole the material contained in this book without obtaining the permission of the author first.

Disclaimer Notice: You must take note that the information in this document is for casual reading and entertainment purpose only. We have made every attempt to provide accurate, up to date and reliable information. We do not express or imply guarantees of any kind. The person who read admit that the writer is not occupied in giving legal, financial, medical, or other advice. We put this book content by sourcing various places.

Please consult a licensed professional before you try any techniques shown in this book.By going through this document, the book lover comes to an agreement that under no situation is the author accountable for any forfeiture, direct or indirect, which they may incur because of the use of material contained in this document, including, but not limited to, - errors, omissions, or inaccuracies.

Thank you!

We hope you enjoyed our book.

As a small family company, your feedback is very important to us .

Please let us know how you like our book at :

pickme.readme@gmail.com

www.ingramcontent.com/pod-product-compliance
Lightning Source LLC
Chambersburg PA
CBHW071418070526
44578CB00003B/597